DR. BARBARA'S 7 DAY TREATMENT FOR DIABETES

Essential guide to dr. Barbara's 21 day juice detox protocol-discover healing and powerful juice recipes to naturally cleanse and detox your whole body for optimal health

Mauricio Andrea

Table of Contents

COPYRIGHT © 2023

CHAPTER ONE

Understanding Diabetes: Causes, Symptoms, and Complications

Introduction: Diabetes is a chronic condition characterized by high levels of glucose (sugar) in the blood. It occurs when the body either doesn't produce enough insulin or can't effectively use the insulin it produces. Insulin is a hormone produced by the pancreas that helps regulate blood sugar levels and allows glucose to enter cells to be used for energy. Understanding the causes, symptoms, and complications of diabetes is crucial for managing the condition effectively and preventing long-term health issues.

Causes of Diabetes: There are several factors that can contribute to the development of diabetes, including genetics, lifestyle choices, and environmental factors. The two main types of diabetes are type 1 and type 2, each with its own set of causes.

Type 1 diabetes is believed to be an autoimmune disorder, where the body's immune system mistakenly attacks and destroys the insulin-producing cells in the pancreas. While the exact cause of this autoimmune response is not fully understood, it is thought to involve a combination of genetic predisposition and environmental triggers, such as viral infections.

Type 2 diabetes, on the other hand, is primarily associated with lifestyle factors such as obesity, physical inactivity, and poor diet. In type 2 diabetes, the body becomes resistant to the effects of insulin, leading to high blood sugar levels. Genetics also play a role in type 2 diabetes, with certain genetic variations increasing the risk of developing the condition.

Other less common types of diabetes include gestational diabetes, which occurs during pregnancy due to hormonal changes that affect insulin sensitivity, and monogenic diabetes, which is caused by mutations in a single gene.

Symptoms of Diabetes: The symptoms of diabetes can vary depending on the type and severity of the condition, but common symptoms include:

- **Frequent urination:** Excess sugar in the blood can cause the kidneys to work harder to filter it out, leading to increased urination.

- **Increased thirst:** The body tries to compensate for fluid loss through frequent urination by increasing thirst.

- **Unexplained weight loss:** When cells don't receive enough glucose for energy, the body starts burning fat and muscle for fuel, leading to weight loss.

- **Fatigue:** Without enough glucose to fuel cells, individuals with diabetes may feel tired and lethargic.

- **Blurred vision:** High blood sugar levels can cause fluid to be pulled from the lenses of the eyes, resulting in blurred vision.

- **Slow wound healing:** Diabetes can affect the body's ability to heal wounds, making cuts and sores take longer to heal.

It's important to note that some people with type 2 diabetes may not experience any symptoms initially, especially in the early stages of the disease. This is why regular screening for diabetes is recommended, especially for individuals with risk factors such as obesity, family history of diabetes, or sedentary lifestyle.

Complications of Diabetes: Untreated or poorly managed diabetes can lead to a range of serious complications affecting various parts of the body. These complications can be acute or chronic and can significantly impact quality of life and life expectancy.

- **Cardiovascular complications:** Diabetes is a major risk factor for cardiovascular diseases such as heart attack, stroke, and peripheral artery disease. High blood sugar levels can damage blood vessels and nerves, increasing the risk of atherosclerosis (hardening and narrowing of the arteries) and blood clots.

- **Nerve damage (neuropathy):** Prolonged high blood sugar levels can damage nerves throughout the body, causing symptoms such as numbness, tingling, pain, and weakness, especially in the extremities. This condition, known as diabetic neuropathy, can lead to serious complications such as foot ulcers and even amputation if left untreated.

- **Kidney damage (nephropathy):** Diabetes is the leading cause of kidney failure, known as diabetic nephropathy. High blood sugar levels over time can damage the small blood vessels in the kidneys, impairing their ability to filter waste products from the blood.

- **Eye damage (retinopathy):** Diabetes can cause damage to the blood vessels in the retina, the light-sensitive tissue at the back of the eye, leading to diabetic retinopathy. This condition can cause vision loss or blindness if left untreated.

- **Foot complications:** Diabetes increases the risk of foot problems due to nerve damage and poor blood circulation. Minor injuries such as cuts, blisters, or sores can become serious infections if not properly treated, potentially leading to amputation.

- **Skin conditions:** People with diabetes are more prone to various skin conditions, including bacterial and fungal infections, as well as diabetic dermopathy (patches of scaly skin).

- **Mental health issues:** Diabetes can have a significant impact on mental health, increasing the risk of depression, anxiety, and diabetes-related distress.

Conclusion: Diabetes is a complex and chronic condition that requires lifelong management to prevent complications and maintain quality of life. Understanding the causes, symptoms, and complications of diabetes is essential for early diagnosis, effective treatment, and appropriate lifestyle modifications. By adopting a healthy lifestyle, monitoring blood sugar levels regularly, and adhering to prescribed treatment plans, individuals with diabetes can minimize their risk of complications and lead fulfilling lives. Regular medical check-ups and consultations with healthcare professionals are crucial for managing diabetes and optimizing overall health and well-being.

CHAPTER TWO

The Role of Herbal Medicine in Managing Diabetes

Diabetes mellitus, a metabolic disorder characterized by elevated blood sugar levels, has become a global health concern due to its increasing prevalence and associated complications. While conventional medications such as insulin and oral hypoglycemic agents remain the cornerstone of diabetes management, there is growing interest in complementary and alternative therapies, including herbal medicine. Herbal remedies have been used for centuries in various cultures to manage diabetes and its related symptoms. This article explores the role of herbal medicine in managing diabetes, including the evidence supporting their use, potential benefits, and safety considerations.

Traditional Herbal Remedies for Diabetes: Throughout history, traditional healers and herbalists have relied on plants and botanical extracts to alleviate the symptoms of diabetes and improve glycemic control. Some of the most commonly used herbs in traditional medicine for diabetes management include:

1. **Bitter Melon (Momordica charantia):** Bitter melon, also known as bitter gourd or karela, is a tropical fruit widely used in Asian cooking and traditional medicine. It contains compounds with hypoglycemic properties, such as charantin, vicine, and polypeptide-p. These compounds help lower

blood sugar levels by increasing insulin secretion, improving insulin sensitivity, and inhibiting glucose absorption in the intestines.

2. **Fenugreek (Trigonella foenum-graecum):** Fenugreek seeds are rich in soluble fiber and saponins, which have been shown to improve glycemic control by delaying carbohydrate digestion and absorption, increasing insulin sensitivity, and enhancing glucose utilization by peripheral tissues.

3. **Ginseng (Panax ginseng, Panax quinquefolius):** Ginseng root has been used in traditional Chinese medicine for its purported anti-diabetic effects. Several studies suggest that ginseng may improve glycemic control by stimulating insulin secretion, enhancing insulin sensitivity, and reducing oxidative stress and inflammation.

4. **Cinnamon (Cinnamomum verum, Cinnamomum cassia):** Cinnamon is a popular spice with antioxidant and anti-inflammatory properties. Some research indicates that cinnamon supplementation may improve fasting blood sugar levels, insulin sensitivity, and lipid profiles in individuals with diabetes.

5. **Gymnema (Gymnemasylvestre):**Gymnema is an herb native to India and has been traditionally used to treat diabetes. It contains compounds called gymnemic acids, which may help lower blood sugar levels by blocking sugar absorption in the

intestines and stimulating insulin secretion from the pancreas.

6. **Aloe Vera (Aloe barbadensis):** Aloe vera gel, derived from the leaves of the aloe plant, has been studied for its potential anti-diabetic properties. Some research suggests that aloe vera supplementation may improve glycemic control and lipid profiles in individuals with type 2 diabetes.

Evidence Supporting Herbal Medicine for Diabetes: While traditional herbal remedies have been used for centuries to manage diabetes, their efficacy and safety have been the subject of scientific investigation in recent years. Several clinical trials and preclinical studies have explored the potential benefits of herbal medicine for diabetes management. Here are some key findings:

1. **Bitter Melon:** Clinical trials have shown that bitter melon supplementation can significantly reduce fasting blood sugar levels and improve glucose tolerance in individuals with type 2 diabetes. However, more research is needed to establish its long-term efficacy and safety.

2. **Fenugreek:** Clinical studies have demonstrated that fenugreek supplementation can improve glycemic control, reduce insulin resistance, and lower fasting blood sugar and HbA1c levels in patients with type 2 diabetes.

3. **Ginseng:** Some clinical trials have reported improvements in fasting blood sugar levels, insulin sensitivity, and HbA1c levels with ginseng supplementation in individuals with type 2 diabetes. However, results have been inconsistent, and further research is warranted.

4. **Cinnamon:** Several meta-analyses have concluded that cinnamon supplementation can modestly reduce fasting blood sugar levels and improve lipid profiles in individuals with type 2 diabetes. However, the clinical significance of these findings remains unclear.

5. **Gymnema:** Clinical studies have shown that gymnema supplementation can lower fasting blood sugar levels, reduce HbA1c levels, and improve insulin sensitivity in patients with type 2 diabetes. However, more high-quality trials are needed to confirm these effects.

6. **Aloe Vera:** Some clinical trials have reported improvements in fasting blood sugar levels, HbA1c levels, and lipid profiles with aloe vera supplementation in individuals with type 2 diabetes. However, additional research is needed to validate these findings and determine the optimal dosage and duration of treatment.

Safety Considerations and Precautions: While herbal remedies may offer potential benefits for diabetes management, it's important to exercise caution and consult with a healthcare professional before using them, especially in conjunction with conventional medications. Some important safety considerations and precautions include:

1. **Potential Interactions:** Herbal remedies can interact with prescription medications, potentially affecting their efficacy or safety. For example, ginseng may interact with anticoagulant drugs, while fenugreek may enhance the hypoglycemic effects of diabetes medications.

2. **Quality and Purity:** The quality and purity of herbal products can vary widely, and contamination with toxins or adulterants is possible. It's essential to choose reputable brands that adhere to quality standards and undergo third-party testing for potency and purity.

3. **Dosage and Formulation:** Herbal remedies are available in various forms, including capsules, tablets, teas, and extracts. It's crucial to follow dosage instructions provided by healthcare professionals or reputable sources and avoid exceeding recommended doses.

4. **Monitoring and Surveillance:** Regular monitoring of blood sugar levels, HbA1c levels, and other relevant parameters is essential for assessing the efficacy and safety of herbal remedies and detecting any adverse effects or interactions.

5. **Contraindications:** Some herbal remedies may be contraindicated in certain populations, such as pregnant or breastfeeding women, individuals with underlying health conditions, or those taking specific medications. It's important to discuss any potential risks with a healthcare professional before using herbal remedies.

Conclusion: Herbal medicine has a long history of use in managing diabetes and may offer potential benefits for glycemic control and related symptoms. While research supporting the efficacy of certain herbs for diabetes management is promising, more high-quality studies are needed to confirm their effects and establish optimal dosing regimens. Additionally, it's essential to exercise caution, consult with a healthcare professional, and integrate herbal remedies into a comprehensive diabetes management plan that includes lifestyle modifications, dietary changes, and conventional medications. By leveraging the therapeutic potential of herbal medicine in a safe and evidence-based manner, individuals with diabetes can enhance their overall health and well-being.

CHAPTER THREE

Preparing for Your Herbal Treatment: Diet and Lifestyle Changes

Embarking on an herbal treatment journey for managing diabetes involves more than just incorporating herbal remedies into your routine; it necessitates comprehensive changes in diet and lifestyle to optimize the efficacy of these natural interventions. While herbal medicine can offer potential benefits in glycemic control and overall health, dietary modifications and lifestyle adjustments play a crucial role in supporting your herbal treatment plan. This article explores the importance of diet and lifestyle changes in preparing for herbal treatment for diabetes and provides practical guidance for integrating these changes into your daily life.

Understanding the Role of Diet and Lifestyle:

Diet and lifestyle factors profoundly influence blood sugar levels, insulin sensitivity, and overall health in individuals with diabetes. By making informed choices about what you eat and how you live, you can complement the effects of herbal remedies and improve your diabetes management outcomes. Here's why diet and lifestyle changes are essential:

1. **Blood Sugar Regulation:** Certain foods can cause rapid spikes in blood sugar levels, leading to unstable glycemic

control. Adopting a balanced diet rich in whole foods, fiber, and nutrients can help stabilize blood sugar levels and reduce the risk of hyperglycemia and hypoglycemia.

2. **Weight Management:** Obesity and excess body weight are significant risk factors for type 2 diabetes and can exacerbate insulin resistance. Making healthy dietary choices and engaging in regular physical activity can support weight loss and improve insulin sensitivity.

3. **Heart Health:** Diabetes increases the risk of cardiovascular diseases such as heart attack and stroke. A heart-healthy diet low in saturated fats, cholesterol, and sodium, combined with regular exercise, can help reduce the risk of cardiovascular complications and promote overall heart health.

4. **Energy Levels and Well-Being:** Diet and lifestyle choices impact energy levels, mood, and overall well-being. Eating nutritious foods and staying physically active can boost energy levels, reduce fatigue, and enhance quality of life in individuals with diabetes.

Key Dietary Recommendations:

1. **Emphasize Whole Foods:** Focus on incorporating whole foods such as fruits, vegetables, whole grains, legumes, nuts, and seeds into your diet. These foods are rich in fiber,

vitamins, minerals, and antioxidants, which support overall health and help stabilize blood sugar levels.

2. **Limit Processed Foods:** Minimize consumption of processed and refined foods high in added sugars, unhealthy fats, and sodium. These foods can contribute to weight gain, insulin resistance, and inflammation, worsening diabetes control.

3. **Control Carbohydrate Intake:** Pay attention to the quantity and quality of carbohydrates in your diet. Choose complex carbohydrates with a low glycemic index, such as whole grains, vegetables, and legumes, which are digested more slowly and have less impact on blood sugar levels.

4. **Moderate Protein Intake:** Include lean sources of protein such as poultry, fish, tofu, legumes, and dairy products in your meals. Protein helps regulate blood sugar levels, promotes satiety, and supports muscle health.

5. **Healthy Fats:** Choose healthy fats such as avocados, nuts, seeds, olive oil, and fatty fish rich in omega-3 fatty acids. These fats have anti-inflammatory properties and can help improve insulin sensitivity and lipid profiles.

6. **Portion Control:** Practice portion control to avoid overeating and maintain a healthy weight. Pay attention to serving sizes and listen to your body's hunger and fullness cues.

Lifestyle Recommendations:

1. **Regular Physical Activity:** Engage in regular exercise, including aerobic activities, strength training, and flexibility exercises. Aim for at least 150 minutes of moderate-intensity aerobic exercise or 75 minutes of vigorous-intensity exercise per week, as recommended by health guidelines.

2. **Stress Management:** Chronic stress can negatively impact blood sugar levels and overall health. Practice stress-reducing techniques such as deep breathing, meditation, yoga, tai chi, or spending time in nature to promote relaxation and well-being.

3. **Adequate Sleep:** Prioritize adequate sleep to support optimal health and glycemic control. Aim for 7-9 hours of quality sleep per night and establish a regular sleep schedule to regulate circadian rhythms.

4. **Hydration:** Stay hydrated by drinking plenty of water throughout the day. Limit consumption of sugary beverages and caffeinated drinks, which can affect blood sugar levels and hydration status.

5. **Regular Monitoring:** Monitor your blood sugar levels regularly as directed by your healthcare provider. Keep track of your dietary choices, physical activity, medication use, and herbal supplementation to identify patterns and make informed adjustments to your diabetes management plan.

Conclusion:

Preparing for herbal treatment for diabetes involves a holistic approach that encompasses dietary modifications, lifestyle adjustments, and herbal supplementation. By adopting a balanced diet rich in whole foods, engaging in regular physical activity, managing stress, prioritizing sleep, and staying hydrated, you can optimize the efficacy of herbal remedies and improve your overall health and well-being. Consult with a healthcare professional or registered dietitian to develop a personalized diabetes management plan that integrates herbal medicine with evidence-based dietary and lifestyle interventions. With dedication, consistency, and support, you can empower yourself to take control of your diabetes and live a healthier, more fulfilling life.

CHAPTER FOUR

Day 1: Introduction to Herbal Remedies for Blood Sugar Control

Welcome to Day 1 of your journey into exploring herbal remedies for blood sugar control. In this introductory session, we will lay the foundation for understanding the role of herbal medicine in managing diabetes, explore some commonly used herbs, and discuss the importance of evidence-based practice in integrating herbal remedies into your diabetes management plan.

Understanding Herbal Medicine for Diabetes:

Herbal medicine, also known as botanical medicine or phytotherapy, involves the use of plant-based remedies to prevent, alleviate, or treat various health conditions, including diabetes. Throughout history, different cultures have relied on the healing properties of plants to manage diabetes symptoms and improve glycemic control. Herbal remedies offer a holistic approach to diabetes management, addressing not only blood sugar levels but also supporting overall health and well-being.

Commonly Used Herbs for Blood Sugar Control:

Several herbs have gained popularity for their potential benefits in regulating blood sugar levels and improving insulin sensitivity. While scientific research on the efficacy of these herbs is ongoing, some commonly used herbs for blood sugar control include:

1. **Bitter Melon (Momordica charantia):** Bitter melon, also known as bitter gourd or karela, is a tropical fruit that has been traditionally used in Asian medicine for its hypoglycemic properties. It contains compounds such as charantin, vicine, and polypeptide-p, which may help lower blood sugar levels by increasing insulin secretion and improving insulin sensitivity.

2. **Fenugreek (Trigonella foenum-graecum):** Fenugreek seeds are rich in soluble fiber and saponins, which have been shown to improve glycemic control by delaying carbohydrate digestion and absorption, enhancing insulin sensitivity, and reducing insulin resistance.

3. **Ginseng (Panax ginseng, Panax quinquefolius):** Ginseng root has been used in traditional Chinese medicine for its purported anti-diabetic effects. Some studies suggest that ginseng may improve insulin sensitivity, enhance glucose utilization, and reduce oxidative stress and inflammation.

4. **Cinnamon (Cinnamomum verum, Cinnamomum cassia):** Cinnamon is a popular spice with antioxidant and anti-inflammatory properties. Research indicates that cinnamon supplementation may improve fasting blood sugar levels, insulin sensitivity, and lipid profiles in individuals with diabetes.

5. **Gymnema (Gymnemasylvestre):**Gymnema is an herb native to India and has been traditionally used to support healthy blood sugar levels. It contains compounds called gymnemic acids, which may help lower blood sugar levels by blocking sugar absorption in the intestines and stimulating insulin secretion from the pancreas.

Importance of Evidence-Based Practice:

While traditional wisdom and anecdotal evidence support the use of herbal remedies for diabetes management, it's essential to approach herbal medicine with a critical mindset and rely on scientific evidence to guide decision-making. Evidence-based practice involves integrating the best available research evidence with clinical expertise and patient preferences to inform treatment decisions.

As you explore herbal remedies for blood sugar control, consider the following principles of evidence-based practice:

1. **Seek Reliable Sources:** Look for information from reputable sources, such as peer-reviewed journals, academic institutions, and government health agencies. Be wary of anecdotal claims or unsupported assertions.

2. **Evaluate Research Studies:** Examine the quality of research studies supporting the use of herbal remedies for diabetes. Consider factors such as study design, sample size, duration, and outcomes measured.

3. **Consult Healthcare Professionals:** Consult with healthcare professionals, such as physicians, registered dietitians, or herbalists, before incorporating herbal remedies into your diabetes management plan. They can provide personalized guidance based on your individual health status, medication regimen, and treatment goals.

4. **Monitor Effectiveness and Safety:** Monitor your blood sugar levels, symptoms, and overall health when using herbal remedies. Pay attention to any changes or adverse reactions and communicate them to your healthcare provider.

Conclusion:

Herbal remedies offer a promising avenue for blood sugar control and diabetes management, but it's crucial to approach them with a well-informed and evidence-based mindset. By understanding the properties of commonly used herbs, evaluating research evidence, and consulting with healthcare professionals, you can make informed decisions about integrating herbal medicine into your diabetes management plan. Stay curious, stay open-minded, and stay committed to optimizing your health and well-being with the power of herbal remedies.

CHAPTER FIVE

Day 2: Herbal Teas and Infusions to Regulate Blood Glucose Levels

Welcome to Day 2 of your exploration into herbal remedies for blood glucose control. Today, we will delve into the world of herbal teas and infusions, discovering how these natural beverages can contribute to regulating blood sugar levels and supporting overall health.

Understanding Herbal Teas and Infusions:

Herbal teas and infusions are beverages made from steeping various parts of plants, including leaves, flowers, roots, and seeds, in hot water. These aromatic and flavorful drinks have been consumed for centuries for their medicinal properties and therapeutic benefits. Herbal teas offer a convenient and enjoyable way to incorporate beneficial herbs into your daily routine, promoting hydration and wellness.

Herbs for Blood Glucose Regulation in Tea Form:

1. **Cinnamon Tea:** Cinnamon, a popular spice with anti-inflammatory and antioxidant properties, is commonly used in herbal teas for blood sugar control. To make cinnamon tea, simply steep a cinnamon stick or ground cinnamon in

hot water for a few minutes. Enjoy this fragrant beverage on its own or with a splash of lemon or honey for added flavor.

2. **Ginger Tea:** Ginger root, known for its warming and digestive properties, may help improve insulin sensitivity and reduce blood sugar levels. To make ginger tea, thinly slice or grate fresh ginger root and steep it in hot water. You can enhance the flavor with a squeeze of lemon or a sprinkle of cinnamon.

3. **Fenugreek Tea:** Fenugreek seeds are rich in soluble fiber and saponins, which have been shown to support healthy blood sugar levels. To make fenugreek tea, soak fenugreek seeds in hot water overnight and strain the liquid in the morning. Drink the infused water as a refreshing herbal tea.

4. **Ginseng Tea:** Ginseng root, prized for its adaptogenic properties, may help improve insulin sensitivity and glucose metabolism. To make ginseng tea, steep sliced ginseng root or ginseng tea bags in hot water for several minutes. Enjoy the earthy flavor of ginseng tea on its own or with a touch of honey.

5. **Hibiscus Tea:** Hibiscus flowers contain polyphenols and antioxidants that may have blood sugar-lowering effects. To make hibiscus tea, steep dried hibiscus flowers in hot water for 5-10 minutes. Serve the vibrant red tea hot or chilled, sweetened with a bit of honey or stevia if desired.

6. **Nettle Tea:** Nettle leaf, a nutrient-rich herb with diuretic properties, may help regulate blood sugar levels and improve overall health. To make nettle tea, steep dried nettle leaves in hot water for 5-10 minutes. Enjoy the earthy and grassy flavor of nettle tea as a nourishing beverage.

Tips for Enjoying Herbal Teas:

1. **Experiment with Flavors:** Mix and match different herbs and spices to create your own custom herbal tea blends. Get creative with combinations such as cinnamon and ginger, hibiscus and rose hips, or nettle and peppermint.

2. **Mindful Brewing:** Pay attention to water temperature and steeping time when brewing herbal teas to extract the optimal flavor and medicinal properties. Follow recommended guidelines for each herb to achieve the desired effects.

3. **Stay Hydrated:** Herbal teas are a great way to stay hydrated throughout the day, especially if you're trying to reduce your consumption of sugary beverages. Keep a variety of herbal teas on hand to enjoy hot or cold, depending on your preference.

4. **Enjoy the Ritual:** Brewing and savoring a cup of herbal tea can be a calming and meditative ritual. Take time to appreciate the aroma, taste, and warmth of your herbal infusion, allowing it to nourish your body and soul.

Conclusion:

Herbal teas and infusions offer a delightful and healthful way to incorporate beneficial herbs into your daily routine. By exploring different herbal teas for blood glucose regulation and experimenting with flavors and combinations, you can discover new favorites while supporting your overall health and well-being. Enjoy the journey of brewing and sipping herbal teas, and embrace the natural healing power of these aromatic beverages. Cheers to good health and vitality!

CHAPTER SIX

Day 3: Incorporating Diabetes-Friendly Herbs into Your Meals

Welcome to Day 3 of your exploration into herbal remedies for managing diabetes. Today, we will focus on incorporating diabetes-friendly herbs into your meals, adding flavor, nutrition, and potential blood sugar benefits to your culinary creations.

Benefits of Using Herbs in Cooking:

Herbs are not only flavorful additions to meals but also offer a wide range of health benefits, including potential blood sugar regulation. By incorporating diabetes-friendly herbs into your cooking, you can enhance the taste of your dishes while promoting better glycemic control and overall wellness.

Diabetes-Friendly Herbs for Cooking:

1. **Basil:** Basil is a fragrant herb commonly used in Mediterranean cuisine. It contains essential oils with antioxidant and anti-inflammatory properties. Add fresh basil leaves to salads, pasta dishes, soups, and sauces for a burst of flavor and health benefits.

2. **Rosemary:** Rosemary is a versatile herb with a distinctive pine-like aroma. It contains rosmarinic acid and other compounds that may help improve insulin sensitivity and

lower blood sugar levels. Use fresh rosemary sprigs to season roasted vegetables, grilled meats, and poultry dishes.

3. **Thyme:** Thyme is a fragrant herb with antibacterial and antioxidant properties. It contains flavonoids and other bioactive compounds that may support blood sugar regulation. Sprinkle fresh thyme leaves over roasted potatoes, soups, stews, and seafood dishes for added flavor and health benefits.

4. **Oregano:** Oregano is a flavorful herb commonly used in Italian and Mediterranean cuisine. It contains compounds such as carvacrol and thymol, which have antioxidant and anti-inflammatory properties. Use dried oregano to season pizza, pasta sauces, roasted vegetables, and grilled meats.

5. **Cilantro (Coriander):** Cilantro, also known as coriander leaf, adds a fresh and citrusy flavor to dishes. It contains antioxidants and bioactive compounds that may help regulate blood sugar levels. Add chopped cilantro leaves to salsas, salads, curries, and stir-fries for a burst of flavor and nutritional benefits.

6. **Parsley:** Parsley is a versatile herb rich in vitamins, minerals, and antioxidants. It contains flavonoids and other phytochemicals that may support blood sugar control. Use fresh parsley leaves as a garnish for soups, salads, pasta dishes, and roasted vegetables.

Tips for Incorporating Herbs into Your Meals:

1. **Use Fresh Herbs Whenever Possible:** Fresh herbs not only provide superior flavor but also retain more of their beneficial nutrients and phytochemicals compared to dried herbs. Grow your own herb garden or purchase fresh herbs from the market for optimal taste and health benefits.

2. **Experiment with Flavor Combinations:** Get creative in the kitchen by experimenting with different herb combinations to elevate the taste of your dishes. Mix and match herbs such as basil, rosemary, and thyme to create unique flavor profiles that complement your favorite recipes.

3. **Add Herbs at the Right Time:** Incorporate fresh herbs into your dishes towards the end of the cooking process to preserve their flavor and aroma. Add delicate herbs like cilantro and parsley just before serving to maximize their freshness and vibrancy.

4. **Enhance Nutritional Content:** Herbs not only enhance the taste of your meals but also contribute valuable nutrients and antioxidants. By incorporating a variety of herbs into your cooking, you can boost the nutritional content of your dishes and support overall health and well-being.

5. **Balance Flavors:** Use herbs to balance the flavors of your dishes by adding depth, freshness, and complexity. Experiment with different herb-to-ingredient ratios to

achieve the perfect balance of flavors and create well-rounded culinary masterpieces.

Conclusion:

Incorporating diabetes-friendly herbs into your meals is a delicious and nutritious way to support blood sugar control and enhance the taste of your dishes. By exploring the diverse world of culinary herbs and experimenting with flavor combinations, you can transform ordinary meals into extraordinary culinary experiences that nourish both body and soul. Get creative in the kitchen, embrace the power of herbs, and enjoy the journey of cooking with flavor and flair!

CHAPTER SEVEN

Day 4: Herbal Supplements and Tinctures for Insulin Sensitivity

Welcome to Day 4 of your journey into herbal remedies for managing diabetes. Today, we will explore herbal supplements and tinctures specifically targeted at improving insulin sensitivity, a key factor in regulating blood sugar levels and managing diabetes effectively.

Understanding Insulin Sensitivity:

Insulin sensitivity refers to how effectively cells respond to insulin, the hormone responsible for regulating blood sugar levels. In individuals with insulin resistance, cells become less responsive to insulin, leading to elevated blood sugar levels and an increased risk of type 2 diabetes. Improving insulin sensitivity is crucial for enhancing glucose uptake by cells and maintaining optimal blood sugar control.

Herbal Supplements for Improving Insulin Sensitivity:

Several herbs have been studied for their potential benefits in improving insulin sensitivity and supporting healthy blood sugar levels. While research on the efficacy of herbal supplements is ongoing, some commonly used herbs for this purpose include:

1. **Berberine:** Berberine is a bioactive compound found in several plants, including goldenseal, barberry, and Oregon grape. Studies suggest that berberine may improve insulin sensitivity, reduce blood sugar levels, and lower HbA1c levels in individuals with type 2 diabetes.

2. **Fenugreek:** Fenugreek seeds are rich in soluble fiber and saponins, which have been shown to enhance insulin sensitivity and improve glycemic control. Fenugreek supplements may help reduce fasting blood sugar levels, postprandial glucose levels, and insulin resistance in individuals with type 2 diabetes.

3. **Cinnamon:** Cinnamon contains bioactive compounds such as cinnamaldehyde and cinnamic acid, which may enhance insulin sensitivity and improve glucose metabolism. Cinnamon supplements have been associated with reductions in fasting blood sugar levels, HbA1c levels, and insulin resistance in individuals with type 2 diabetes.

4. **Alpha-Lipoic Acid (ALA):** Alpha-lipoic acid is a powerful antioxidant that plays a role in energy metabolism and glucose utilization. ALA supplements may improve insulin sensitivity, reduce oxidative stress, and enhance glucose uptake in skeletal muscle cells, potentially benefiting individuals with insulin resistance and type 2 diabetes.

5. **Gymnema:**Gymnema leaf extracts contain bioactive compounds called gymnemic acids, which may help improve insulin sensitivity and promote glucose uptake by cells. Gymnema supplements have been shown to reduce fasting blood sugar levels, HbA1c levels, and insulin resistance in individuals with type 2 diabetes.

Herbal Tinctures for Improving Insulin Sensitivity:

Tinctures are concentrated liquid extracts of herbs, typically made by soaking plant material in alcohol or glycerin to extract their active constituents. While herbal tinctures are less commonly studied than supplements, they offer a convenient and potent way to consume medicinal herbs for improving insulin sensitivity. Some herbs commonly used in tincture form for this purpose include:

1. **Ginseng:** Ginseng root, available in tincture form, has been traditionally used to support healthy blood sugar levels and improve insulin sensitivity. Ginseng tinctures can be added to water or herbal teas for easy consumption.

2. **Holy Basil (Tulsi):** Holy basil, revered for its adaptogenic properties, may help enhance insulin sensitivity and reduce blood sugar levels. Holy basil tinctures can be taken orally or added to beverages for a refreshing herbal boost.

3. **Milk Thistle:** Milk thistle is a liver-supportive herb that may benefit individuals with insulin resistance by improving liver function and reducing inflammation. Milk thistle tinctures can be consumed alone or added to juices or smoothies for a nutritional boost.

4. **Bitter Melon:** Bitter melon tinctures contain bioactive compounds with potential blood sugar-lowering effects. Bitter melon tinctures can be diluted in water or mixed with other herbal tinctures for a synergistic blend.

Precautions and Considerations:

Before incorporating herbal supplements or tinctures into your diabetes management plan, it's essential to consider the following precautions:

1. **Consult Healthcare Professional:** Consult with a healthcare professional, such as a physician or herbalist, before starting any new herbal supplement or tincture, especially if you have underlying health conditions or are taking medications.

2. **Monitor Blood Sugar Levels:** Regularly monitor your blood sugar levels when using herbal supplements or tinctures to assess their effects on glycemic control. Keep track of any changes in blood sugar levels and communicate them to your healthcare provider.

3. **Start Slowly:** Start with a low dose of herbal supplements or tinctures and gradually increase the dosage as tolerated. Pay attention to any adverse reactions or side effects and adjust your dosage accordingly.

4. **Quality and Purity:** Choose high-quality herbal supplements and tinctures from reputable brands that undergo third-party testing for potency and purity. Avoid products containing fillers, additives, or contaminants.

Conclusion:

Herbal supplements and tinctures offer promising avenues for improving insulin sensitivity and supporting healthy blood sugar levels in individuals with diabetes. By exploring the potential benefits of herbs such as berberine, fenugreek, cinnamon, and ginseng, you can complement your diabetes management plan with natural and holistic interventions. Remember to consult with a healthcare professional, monitor your blood sugar levels, and prioritize high-quality herbal products for optimal safety and efficacy. With careful consideration and informed decision-making, you can harness the power of herbal medicine to enhance your overall health and well-being.

CHAPTER EIGHT

Day 5: Stress Management and Herbal Remedies for Diabetes-Related Stress

Welcome to Day 5 of your exploration into herbal remedies for managing diabetes. Today, we will focus on stress management and how herbal remedies can help alleviate diabetes-related stress, a common concern for individuals living with this condition.

Understanding Diabetes-Related Stress:

Living with diabetes can be challenging, as it requires constant monitoring of blood sugar levels, adherence to dietary and lifestyle changes, and the management of potential complications. Diabetes-related stress refers to the emotional and psychological burden experienced by individuals with diabetes due to the demands of self-care, fear of complications, and concerns about the future.

The Impact of Stress on Diabetes:

Stress can have a significant impact on diabetes management and overall health. Chronic stress can lead to elevated blood sugar levels, insulin resistance, and poor glycemic control in individuals with diabetes. Additionally, stress hormones such as cortisol and adrenaline can interfere with insulin action, increase appetite, and promote unhealthy behaviors such as overeating and sedentary lifestyle choices.

Herbal Remedies for Stress Management:

Several herbs have adaptogenic properties, meaning they help the body adapt to stress and promote a sense of balance and well-being. By incorporating these herbal remedies into your routine, you can support your body's natural response to stress and mitigate the negative effects of diabetes-related stress on your health. Some herbs commonly used for stress management include:

1. **Ashwagandha (Withaniasomnifera):** Ashwagandha is an adaptogenic herb traditionally used in Ayurvedic medicine to reduce stress and promote relaxation. Studies suggest that ashwagandha supplementation may lower cortisol levels, improve mood, and enhance resilience to stress.

2. **Rhodiola (Rhodiola rosea):** Rhodiola is an adaptogenic herb known for its stress-relieving properties. Rhodiola supplementation may help reduce symptoms of stress, fatigue, and anxiety, while improving cognitive function and overall well-being.

3. **Holy Basil (Tulsi):** Holy basil is revered in Ayurvedic medicine for its adaptogenic and antioxidant properties. Holy basil supplementation may help reduce stress, anxiety, and

depression, while supporting healthy blood sugar levels and cardiovascular function.

4. **Lemon Balm (Melissa officinalis):** Lemon balm is a calming herb that may help reduce stress, anxiety, and insomnia. Lemon balm supplementation or tea consumption can promote relaxation and improve mood in individuals with diabetes-related stress.

5. **Chamomile (Matricaria chamomilla):** Chamomile is a soothing herb with sedative properties that can help reduce stress and promote better sleep. Chamomile tea is a popular natural remedy for relaxation and stress relief.

Incorporating Herbal Remedies into Your Routine:

1. **Herbal Teas:** Brew herbal teas using stress-relieving herbs such as ashwagandha, rhodiola, holy basil, lemon balm, or chamomile. Enjoy a cup of herbal tea in the morning or evening as part of your self-care routine.

2. **Herbal Supplements:** Consider taking herbal supplements containing stress-relieving herbs to support your body's response to stress. Choose high-quality products from reputable brands and follow recommended dosage guidelines.

3. **Aromatherapy:** Use essential oils derived from stress-relieving herbs, such as lavender, bergamot, or frankincense,

in aromatherapy diffusers or massage oils to promote relaxation and reduce stress.

4. **Herbal Baths:** Add dried herbs such as lavender, chamomile, or lemon balm to your bathwater to create a soothing herbal bath experience. Allow the aromatic herbs to infuse the water and envelop you in relaxation.

5. **Mind-Body Practices:** Combine herbal remedies with mind-body practices such as meditation, deep breathing exercises, yoga, or tai chi to enhance stress management and promote overall well-being.

Conclusion:

Managing diabetes-related stress is essential for optimizing glycemic control and overall health. By incorporating herbal remedies with adaptogenic properties into your routine, you can support your body's natural response to stress, promote relaxation, and enhance your ability to cope with the challenges of living with diabetes. Experiment with different herbal remedies, find what works best for you, and prioritize self-care practices that nurture your mind, body, and spirit. With a holistic approach to stress management, you can cultivate resilience, balance, and vitality on your diabetes journey.

CHAPTER NINE

Day 6: Physical Activity and Exercise Guidelines for Diabetes Management

Welcome to Day 6 of your journey into managing diabetes through holistic approaches. Today, we'll focus on the importance of physical activity and exercise in diabetes management and explore practical guidelines for incorporating movement into your daily routine.

Understanding the Benefits of Physical Activity:

Physical activity plays a crucial role in diabetes management by improving insulin sensitivity, lowering blood sugar levels, and reducing the risk of cardiovascular complications. Regular exercise can also help control weight, improve mood, boost energy levels, and enhance overall well-being.

Exercise Guidelines for Individuals with Diabetes:

1. **Types of Exercise:** Incorporate a combination of aerobic exercise, strength training, and flexibility exercises into your routine for comprehensive health benefits. Aim for a variety of activities, such as brisk walking, cycling, swimming, resistance training, yoga, or Pilates.

2. **Duration:** Strive for at least 150 minutes of moderate-intensity aerobic exercise per week, spread across several

days. Alternatively, aim for 75 minutes of vigorous-intensity aerobic exercise per week. Include strength training exercises targeting major muscle groups at least two days per week.

3. **Intensity:** Moderate-intensity aerobic exercise should elevate your heart rate and breathing, making it challenging to hold a conversation but still possible. Vigorous-intensity aerobic exercise will significantly increase your heart rate and breathing, making it difficult to speak more than a few words without pausing for breath.

4. **Frequency:** Aim for regular physical activity most days of the week, aiming for consistency rather than sporadic intense sessions. If you're just starting, begin with shorter sessions and gradually increase duration and intensity as your fitness improves.

5. **Progression:** Gradually increase the duration, intensity, and frequency of your exercise sessions over time to challenge your body and improve fitness levels. Listen to your body and adjust your routine as needed to prevent injury and avoid burnout.

6. **Safety Considerations:** Before starting a new exercise program, consult with your healthcare provider to ensure it's safe for you, especially if you have underlying health conditions or complications related to diabetes. Consider

working with a certified fitness professional or exercise physiologist to develop a personalized exercise plan tailored to your needs and goals.

Incorporating Physical Activity into Your Routine:

1. **Set Realistic Goals:** Establish achievable goals for physical activity based on your current fitness level, health status, and lifestyle. Start with small, manageable steps and gradually increase activity as you build confidence and stamina.

2. **Find Activities You Enjoy:** Choose physical activities that you enjoy and look forward to, whether it's dancing, hiking, gardening, or playing sports. The key is to make exercise enjoyable and sustainable for the long term.

3. **Make It Social:** Invite friends, family members, or coworkers to join you in physical activities for added motivation and accountability. Consider joining exercise classes, sports leagues, or community fitness groups to connect with like-minded individuals and make new friends.

4. **Schedule It:** Treat physical activity like any other important appointment and schedule it into your calendar. Find time slots that work best for you, whether it's early morning,

during lunch breaks, or in the evening, and stick to your schedule as much as possible.

5. **Break It Up:** If you have difficulty finding large blocks of time for exercise, break your activity into smaller, more manageable segments throughout the day. Even short bursts of activity, such as a brisk 10-minute walk after meals, can add up to significant health benefits over time.

Conclusion:

Physical activity is a cornerstone of diabetes management, offering numerous benefits for both physical and mental health. By following exercise guidelines, incorporating movement into your daily routine, and making physical activity enjoyable and sustainable, you can improve glycemic control, reduce the risk of complications, and enhance overall well-being. Remember to consult with your healthcare provider before starting a new exercise program, prioritize safety, and listen to your body's signals as you embark on your journey toward a healthier, more active lifestyle. With dedication, consistency, and support, you can reap the rewards of regular physical activity and live well with diabetes.

CHAPTER TEN

Day 7: Reflecting on Your Treatment Progress and Creating a Long-Term Plan

Congratulations on completing seven days of exploring holistic approaches to managing diabetes! As we conclude this journey, it's essential to take time to reflect on your treatment progress, celebrate your achievements, and create a long-term plan for continued success in managing diabetes.

Reflecting on Your Treatment Progress:

1. **Assess Your Goals:** Reflect on the goals you set at the beginning of this journey. Have you made progress toward achieving them? Celebrate your accomplishments, no matter how small, and acknowledge the effort you've put into improving your health.

2. **Evaluate Your Strategies:** Consider the holistic approaches you've explored, including herbal remedies, dietary changes, physical activity, stress management techniques, and lifestyle modifications. Which strategies have been most effective for you? Which ones have been more challenging to implement?

3. **Monitor Your Health:** Pay attention to changes in your blood sugar levels, energy levels, mood, weight, and overall well-being since incorporating holistic treatments into your

diabetes management plan. Keep track of any improvements or setbacks and consider how they may relate to your lifestyle choices.

Creating a Long-Term Plan:

1. **Set Realistic Goals:** Based on your reflections, establish new goals or refine existing ones for your long-term diabetes management plan. Make sure your goals are specific, measurable, achievable, relevant, and time-bound (SMART) to keep you motivated and on track.

2. **Develop a Sustainable Routine:** Identify the holistic approaches that have been most beneficial for you and incorporate them into a sustainable daily routine. Consider how you can integrate herbal remedies, healthy eating habits, regular physical activity, stress management techniques, and self-care practices into your lifestyle in the long term.

3. **Seek Continuous Learning:** Stay informed about the latest research, trends, and developments in diabetes management and holistic health practices. Keep an open mind and be willing to explore new ideas, treatments, and approaches that may benefit your health and well-being.

4. **Build a Support Network:** Surround yourself with supportive friends, family members, healthcare providers, and community resources that can offer encouragement,

guidance, and accountability on your diabetes journey. Consider joining support groups, online forums, or social media communities where you can connect with others facing similar challenges and share experiences and insights.

5. **Regularly Review and Adjust:** Schedule regular check-ins with yourself to review your progress, reassess your goals, and make any necessary adjustments to your treatment plan. Be flexible and adaptive as you navigate the ups and downs of managing diabetes, and don't hesitate to seek professional guidance when needed.

Conclusion:

As you reflect on your treatment progress and create a long-term plan for managing diabetes, remember that you are in control of your health and well-being. By integrating holistic approaches into your daily life, setting realistic goals, developing sustainable routines, seeking continuous learning, building a support network, and regularly reviewing and adjusting your plan, you can empower yourself to live well with diabetes and thrive in the years to come. Celebrate your achievements, stay committed to your health goals, and embrace the journey of self-discovery and growth. With determination, resilience, and a positive mindset, you can overcome challenges, achieve success, and live a vibrant and fulfilling life with diabetes.

Herban Iron:

BONUS: SOME HERBAL REMEDIES FOR HEALTH AND WELLNESS

Definition: Herban Iron is a dietary supplement designed to provide an easily absorbable form of iron to support healthy iron levels in the body. It's particularly beneficial for individuals with iron deficiency or anemia.

Ingredients: Herban Iron typically contains iron in the form of ferrous bisglycinate, which is a highly bioavailable and gentle form of iron that is less likely to cause digestive upset or constipation compared to other forms of iron. It may also contain other ingredients such as vitamin C to enhance iron absorption.

How to Prepare: Herban Iron is usually available in capsule or liquid form. Capsules are taken orally with water, while liquid forms may be mixed with water or juice before consumption. It's important to follow the recommended dosage on the product label.

Dosage: The appropriate dosage of Herban Iron depends on factors such as age, gender, and the severity of iron deficiency. It's important to consult with a healthcare professional to determine the correct dosage for individual needs.

How to Use: Herban Iron capsules are typically taken orally with water, while liquid forms may be mixed with water or juice before consumption. It's important to take Herban Iron as directed and to avoid taking it with dairy products, antacids, or other substances that may interfere with iron absorption.

Side Effects: While Herban Iron is generally considered safe for most people when used as directed, some individuals may experience mild side effects such as gastrointestinal discomfort or constipation. It's important to consult with a healthcare professional before starting any new supplement regimen, especially if you have underlying health conditions or are taking medications.

Manjakani:

Definition: Manjakani, also known as Quercus infectoria or oak gall, is a natural substance derived from the oak tree. It has been used for centuries in traditional medicine for its potential health benefits, particularly for women's health and vaginal tightening.

Ingredients: Manjakani contains various bioactive compounds, including tannins, flavonoids, and gallic acid. These compounds are believed to contribute to the herb's medicinal properties, including its potential as an astringent and antiseptic agent.

How to Prepare: Manjakani is typically available in powder, capsule, or liquid extract form. It can be taken orally or used topically depending on the intended use. For vaginal tightening, manjakani may be applied topically as a gel or inserted into the vagina in capsule form.

Dosage: The appropriate dosage of manjakani can vary depending on factors such as age, health status, and the specific preparation being used. It's important to follow the recommended dosage on the product label or consult with a qualified herbalist or healthcare professional for personalized guidance.

How to Use: Manjakani can be taken orally or used topically depending on the intended use. It's important to use manjakani products as directed and to discontinue use if any adverse effects occur.

Side Effects: Manjakani is generally considered safe for most people when used in moderate amounts. However, some individuals may experience allergic reactions or skin irritation when used topically. It's important to use manjakani under the guidance of a healthcare professional and to discontinue use if any adverse effects occur.

Red Clover:

Definition: Red clover, scientifically known as Trifolium pratense, is a flowering plant belonging to the legume family. It's native to Europe, Western Asia, and Northwest Africa but has been naturalized in many other regions. Red clover has been used in traditional medicine for various purposes, including its potential to support women's health and menopausal symptoms.

Ingredients: Red clover contains several bioactive compounds, including isoflavones (such as genistein and daidzein), flavonoids, and phytoestrogens. These compounds are believed to contribute to the herb's medicinal properties, including its potential as a hormone-balancing agent and its ability to support cardiovascular health.

How to Prepare: Red clover is typically prepared and consumed as an herbal tea or tincture. To make tea, dried red clover flowers are steeped in hot water for several minutes before being strained and consumed. Tinctures are prepared by steeping the flowers in alcohol or vinegar to extract their active compounds.

Dosage: The appropriate dosage of red clover can vary depending on factors such as age, health status, and the specific preparation being used. It's important to follow the recommended dosage on the product label or consult with a qualified herbalist or healthcare professional for personalized guidance.

How to Use: Red clover tea or tincture is typically taken orally. It's important to use red clover products as directed and to discontinue use if any adverse effects occur.

Side Effects: Red clover is generally considered safe for most people when used in moderate amounts. However, some individuals may experience allergic reactions or digestive upset. It may also interact with certain medications or have adverse effects in individuals with certain health conditions. It's important to use red clover under the guidance of a healthcare professional and to discontinue use if any adverse effects occur.

Red Raspberry:

Definition: Red raspberry, scientifically known as Rubus idaeus, is a species of raspberry native to Europe and northern Asia. It's widely cultivated for its delicious berries and has been used in traditional medicine for various purposes, including its potential to support women's health during pregnancy and childbirth.

Ingredients: Red raspberry contains several bioactive compounds, including flavonoids, ellagic acid, anthocyanins, and vitamin C. These compounds are believed to contribute to the herb's medicinal properties, including its potential as an antioxidant, anti-inflammatory, and uterine tonic.

How to Prepare: Red raspberry leaf is typically prepared and consumed as an herbal tea or infusion. To make tea, dried red raspberry leaves are steeped in hot water for several minutes before being strained and consumed.

Dosage: The appropriate dosage of red raspberry leaf can vary depending on factors such as age, health status, and the specific preparation being used. It's important to follow the recommended dosage on the product label or consult with a qualified herbalist or healthcare professional for personalized guidance.

How to Use: Red raspberry leaf tea is typically taken orally. It's often recommended for pregnant individuals in the later stages of pregnancy to support uterine health and prepare for childbirth. It's important to use red raspberry leaf products as directed and to discontinue use if any adverse effects occur.

Side Effects: Red raspberry leaf is generally considered safe for most people when used in moderate amounts. However, some individuals may experience allergic reactions or digestive upset. Pregnant individuals should consult with a healthcare professional before using red raspberry leaf, especially if they have any underlying health conditions or are taking medications. It's important to use red raspberry leaf under the guidance of a healthcare professional and to discontinue use if any adverse effects occur.

Rhubarb:

Definition: Rhubarb, scientifically known as Rheum rhabarbarum, is a perennial plant cultivated for its edible stalks. While primarily used in culinary applications, rhubarb has also been utilized in traditional medicine for its potential health benefits, particularly for digestive health.

Ingredients: Rhubarb stalks contain various bioactive compounds, including anthraquinones (such as emodin and rhein), fiber, vitamins (such as vitamin K), and minerals (including calcium and potassium). These compounds are believed to contribute to the herb's medicinal properties, including its potential as a laxative and digestive aid.

How to Prepare: Rhubarb stalks are typically cooked before consumption, as the raw stalks are very tart and can be unpleasant to eat. They are often used in pies, crisps, jams, sauces, and other desserts, as well as in savory dishes. Rhubarb can also be used to make compotes, jams, and preserves.

Dosage: There is no specific dosage for rhubarb in culinary applications, as it is used as a food rather than a medicinal herb. However, when used for its potential laxative effects, it's important to consume rhubarb in moderation to avoid gastrointestinal upset.

How to Use: Rhubarb stalks can be chopped and cooked in various dishes, including pies, sauces, and jams. It's important to remove and discard the leaves, as they contain toxic compounds. When using rhubarb for its potential laxative effects, it's typically consumed as part of a cooked dish or in the form of a rhubarb-based herbal remedy.

Side Effects: Rhubarb stalks are generally safe for most people when consumed in moderate amounts as part of a balanced diet. However, excessive intake may lead to digestive upset or adverse effects due to the presence of oxalic acid, which can bind to calcium and form kidney stones in susceptible individuals. It's important to use rhubarb in moderation and to consult with a healthcare professional if you have any concerns or underlying health conditions.

Sarsaparilla:

Definition: Sarsaparilla refers to several species of plants belonging to the Smilax genus, including Smilax regelii and Smilax officinalis. It has been used historically in traditional medicine for its potential health benefits, particularly for its purported detoxifying and anti-inflammatory properties.

Ingredients: Sarsaparilla contains various bioactive compounds, including saponins (such as sarsaponin and smilagenin), flavonoids, phenolic acids, and sterols. These compounds are believed to contribute to the herb's medicinal properties, including its potential as a diuretic, blood purifier, and anti-inflammatory agent.

How to Prepare: Sarsaparilla root is typically prepared and consumed as an herbal tea, decoction, or tincture. To make tea, dried sarsaparilla root is steeped in hot water for several minutes before being strained and consumed. Decoctions involve boiling the root in water to extract its active compounds, while tinctures are prepared by steeping the root in alcohol or vinegar.

Dosage: The appropriate dosage of sarsaparilla can vary depending on factors such as age, health status, and the specific preparation being used. It's important to follow the recommended dosage on the product label or consult with a qualified herbalist or healthcare professional for personalized guidance.

How to Use: Sarsaparilla tea or tincture is typically taken orally. It's important to use sarsaparilla products as directed and to discontinue use if any adverse effects occur.

Side Effects: Sarsaparilla is generally considered safe for most people when used in moderate amounts. However, some individuals may experience allergic reactions or digestive upset. It may also interact with certain medications or have adverse effects in individuals with certain health conditions. It's important to use sarsaparilla under the guidance of a healthcare professional and to discontinue use if any adverse effects occur.

Tila:

Definition: Tila, also known as linden flower or lime blossom, refers to the flowers of the Tilia genus, primarily Tilia europaea and Tilia cordata. These trees are native to Europe, but they are also cultivated in other regions for their fragrant and medicinal flowers.

Ingredients: Tila flowers contain various bioactive compounds, including flavonoids, phenolic acids, and volatile oils. These compounds are believed to contribute to the herb's medicinal properties, including its potential as a mild sedative, anxiolytic, and anti-inflammatory agent.

How to Prepare: Tila flowers are typically prepared and consumed as an herbal tea or infusion. To make tea, dried tila flowers are steeped in hot water for several minutes before being strained and consumed.

Dosage: The appropriate dosage of tila can vary depending on factors such as age, health status, and the specific preparation being used. It's important to follow the recommended dosage on the product label or consult with a qualified herbalist or healthcare professional for personalized guidance.

How to Use: Tila tea is typically taken orally. It's often consumed in the evening as a calming bedtime beverage or during times of stress or anxiety. It's important to use tila products as directed and to discontinue use if any adverse effects occur.

Side Effects: Tila is generally considered safe for most people when used in moderate amounts. However, some individuals may experience allergic reactions or digestive upset. It may also interact with certain medications or have adverse effects in individuals with certain health conditions. It's important to use tila under the guidance of a healthcare professional and to discontinue use if any adverse effects occur.

Valerian:

Definition: Valerian, scientifically known as Valeriana officinalis, is a perennial flowering plant native to Europe and Asia. It has been used for centuries in traditional medicine for its potential calming and sedative effects.

Ingredients: Valerian root contains several bioactive compounds, including valerenic acid, valepotriates, and volatile oils. These compounds are believed to contribute to the herb's medicinal properties, including its potential as a sedative, anxiolytic, and sleep aid.

How to Prepare: Valerian root is typically prepared and consumed as an herbal tea, tincture, or capsule. To make tea, dried valerian root is steeped in hot water for several minutes before being strained and consumed. Tinctures are prepared by steeping the root in alcohol or vinegar to extract its active compounds.

Dosage: The appropriate dosage of valerian can vary depending on factors such as age, health status, and the specific preparation being used. It's important to follow the recommended dosage on the product label or consult with a qualified herbalist or healthcare professional for personalized guidance.

How to Use: Valerian tea, tincture, or capsules are typically taken orally. It's often consumed in the evening as a sleep aid or during times of stress or anxiety. It's important to use valerian products as directed and to discontinue use if any adverse effects occur.

Side Effects: Valerian is generally considered safe for most people when used in moderate amounts. However, some individuals may experience mild side effects such as drowsiness, headache, or gastrointestinal upset. It may also interact with certain medications or have adverse effects in individuals with certain health conditions. It's important to use valerian under the guidance of a healthcare professional and to discontinue use if any adverse effects occur.

Wild Cherry Bark:

Definition: Wild cherry bark, scientifically known as Prunus serotina, is the bark obtained from the black cherry tree native to North America. It has been used traditionally in Native American and folk medicine for its potential health benefits, particularly for respiratory and digestive issues.

Ingredients: Wild cherry bark contains various bioactive compounds, including cyanogenic glycosides (such as prunasin and amygdalin), flavonoids, and phenolic acids. These compounds are believed to contribute to the herb's medicinal properties, including its potential as an expectorant, cough suppressant, and mild sedative.

How to Prepare: Wild cherry bark is typically prepared and consumed as an herbal tea, decoction, or syrup. To make tea, dried wild cherry bark is steeped in hot water for several minutes before being strained and consumed. Decoctions involve boiling the bark in water to extract its active compounds, while syrups are made by simmering the bark with sugar or honey to create a thick, sweet liquid.

Dosage: The appropriate dosage of wild cherry bark can vary depending on factors such as age, health status, and the specific preparation being used. It's important to follow the recommended dosage on the product label or consult with a qualified herbalist or healthcare professional for personalized guidance.

How to Use: Wild cherry bark tea, decoction, or syrup is typically taken orally. It's often consumed to soothe coughs, sore throats, and other respiratory symptoms. It's important to use wild cherry bark products as directed and to discontinue use if any adverse effects occur.

Side Effects: Wild cherry bark is generally considered safe for most people when used in moderate amounts. However, it contains cyanogenic glycosides, which can release cyanide in the body when metabolized. While the risk of cyanide poisoning from consuming wild cherry bark is low when used appropriately, excessive intake or prolonged use may lead to adverse effects. It's important to use wild cherry bark under the guidance of a healthcare professional and to discontinue use if any adverse effects occur.

Yellowdock:

Definition: Yellowdock, scientifically known as Rumex crispus, is a perennial flowering plant native to Europe and western Asia but is also found in North America. It has a long history of use in traditional medicine, particularly among Indigenous peoples, for its potential health benefits.

Ingredients: Yellowdock root contains various bioactive compounds, including anthraquinone glycosides (such as emodin and chrysophanol), tannins, and vitamins (including vitamin A and vitamin C). These compounds are believed to contribute to the herb's medicinal properties, including its potential as a laxative, blood cleanser, and liver tonic.

How to Prepare: Yellowdock root is typically prepared and consumed as an herbal tea, tincture, or capsule. To make tea, dried yellowdock root is steeped in hot water for several minutes before being strained and consumed. Tinctures are prepared by steeping the root in alcohol or vinegar to extract its active compounds.

Dosage: The appropriate dosage of yellowdock can vary depending on factors such as age, health status, and the specific preparation being used. It's important to follow the recommended dosage on the product label or consult with a qualified herbalist or healthcare professional for personalized guidance.

How to Use: Yellowdock tea, tincture, or capsules are typically taken orally. It's often consumed to support digestion, promote bowel regularity, and cleanse the blood. It's important to use yellowdock products as directed and to discontinue use if any adverse effects occur.

Side Effects: Yellowdock is generally considered safe for most people when used in moderate amounts. However, some individuals may experience mild side effects such as gastrointestinal upset or allergic reactions. It may also interact with certain medications or have adverse effects in individuals with certain health conditions. It's important to use yellowdock under the guidance of a healthcare professional and to discontinue use if any adverse effects occur.

Yellowdock Root:

Definition: Yellowdock root, scientifically known as Rumex crispus, is the root of a perennial flowering plant native to Europe and western Asia, also found in North America. It has a long history of use in traditional medicine, particularly among Indigenous peoples, for its potential health benefits.

Ingredients: Yellowdock root contains various bioactive compounds, including anthraquinone glycosides (such as emodin and chrysophanol), tannins, and vitamins (including vitamin A and vitamin C). These compounds are believed to contribute to the herb's medicinal properties, including its potential as a laxative, blood cleanser, and liver tonic.

How to Prepare: Yellowdock root is typically prepared and consumed as an herbal tea, tincture, or capsule. To make tea, dried yellowdock root is steeped in hot water for several minutes before being strained and consumed. Tinctures are prepared by steeping the root in alcohol or vinegar to extract its active compounds.

Dosage: The appropriate dosage of yellowdock root can vary depending on factors such as age, health status, and the specific preparation being used. It's important to follow the recommended dosage on the product label or consult with a qualified herbalist or healthcare professional for personalized guidance.

How to Use: Yellowdock root tea, tincture, or capsules are typically taken orally. It's often consumed to support digestion, promote bowel regularity, and cleanse the blood. It's important to use yellowdock root products as directed and to discontinue use if any adverse effects occur.

Side Effects: Yellowdock root is generally considered safe for most people when used in moderate amounts. However, some individuals may experience mild side effects such as gastrointestinal upset or allergic reactions. It may also interact with certain medications or have adverse effects in individuals with certain health conditions. It's important to use yellowdock root under the guidance of a healthcare professional and to discontinue use if any adverse effects occur.

Agrimony:

Definition: Agrimony, scientifically known as Agrimonia eupatoria, is a perennial herbaceous plant native to Europe, Asia, and North America. It has a long history of use in traditional medicine, particularly in European folk medicine, for its potential health benefits.

Ingredients: Agrimony contains various bioactive compounds, including tannins, flavonoids, phenolic acids, and volatile oils. These compounds are believed to contribute to the herb's medicinal properties, including its potential as an astringent, anti-inflammatory, and digestive aid.

How to Prepare: Agrimony is typically prepared and consumed as an herbal tea, tincture, or poultice. To make tea, dried agrimony leaves and flowers are steeped in hot water for several minutes before being strained and consumed. Tinctures are prepared by steeping the herb in alcohol or vinegar to extract its active compounds.

Dosage: The appropriate dosage of agrimony can vary depending on factors such as age, health status, and the specific preparation being used. It's important to follow the recommended dosage on the product label or consult with a qualified herbalist or healthcare professional for personalized guidance.

How to Use: Agrimony tea, tincture, or poultice is typically taken orally or applied topically. It's often consumed to soothe gastrointestinal issues, such as indigestion and diarrhea, or used externally to treat skin conditions.

Side Effects: Agrimony is generally considered safe for most people when used in moderate amounts. However, some individuals may experience allergic reactions or gastrointestinal upset. It may also interact with certain medications or have adverse effects in individuals with certain health conditions. It's important to use agrimony under the guidance of a healthcare professional and to discontinue use if any adverse effects occur.

Alfalfa:

Definition: Alfalfa, scientifically known as Medicago sativa, is a flowering plant in the pea family native to Asia but cultivated worldwide. It's primarily grown as fodder for livestock, but it has also been used in traditional medicine for its potential health benefits.

Ingredients: Alfalfa contains various bioactive compounds, including vitamins (such as vitamin A, vitamin C, and vitamin K), minerals (including calcium, magnesium, and potassium), amino acids, and phytoestrogens. These compounds are believed to contribute to the herb's medicinal properties, including its potential as a nutritive tonic, diuretic, and hormone balancer.

How to Prepare: Alfalfa is typically consumed as sprouts, herbal tea, or in supplement form (such as capsules or tablets). To make tea, dried alfalfa leaves are steeped in hot water for several minutes before being strained and consumed.

Dosage: The appropriate dosage of alfalfa can vary depending on factors such as age, health status, and the specific preparation being used. It's important to follow the recommended dosage on the product label or consult with a qualified herbalist or healthcare professional for personalized guidance.

How to Use: Alfalfa sprouts, tea, or supplements are typically taken orally. It's often consumed as a dietary supplement to support overall health and well-being, as well as to promote kidney health and hormone balance.

Side Effects: Alfalfa is generally considered safe for most people when consumed in moderate amounts. However, some individuals may experience allergic reactions or digestive upset. It may also interact with certain medications or have adverse effects in individuals with certain health conditions, such as autoimmune diseases or hormone-sensitive conditions. Pregnant or breastfeeding individuals should consult with a healthcare professional before using alfalfa supplements. It's important to use alfalfa under the guidance of a healthcare professional and to discontinue use if any adverse effects occur.

Ashwagandha:

Definition: Ashwagandha, scientifically known as Withaniasomnifera, is a small shrub native to India, the Middle East, and parts of Africa. It has a long history of use in Ayurvedic medicine for its potential health benefits, particularly for its adaptogenic properties.

Ingredients: Ashwagandha root contains various bioactive compounds, including alkaloids (such as withanolides), steroidal lactones, and flavonoids. These compounds are believed to contribute to the herb's medicinal properties, including its potential as an adaptogen, anti-inflammatory, and immune-modulating agent.

How to Prepare: Ashwagandha is typically consumed as a powdered root, herbal tea, tincture, or in supplement form (such as capsules or tablets). To make tea, dried ashwagandha root is steeped in hot water for several minutes before being strained and consumed.

Dosage: The appropriate dosage of ashwagandha can vary depending on factors such as age, health status, and the specific preparation being used. It's important to follow the recommended dosage on the product label or consult with a qualified herbalist or healthcare professional for personalized guidance.

How to Use: Ashwagandha powder, tea, tincture, or supplements are typically taken orally. It's often consumed to support stress management, promote relaxation, and boost overall vitality and well-being.

Side Effects: Ashwagandha is generally considered safe for most people when used in moderate amounts. However, some individuals may experience mild side effects such as gastrointestinal upset or drowsiness. It may also interact with certain medications or have adverse effects in individuals with certain health conditions, such as autoimmune diseases or thyroid disorders. Pregnant or breastfeeding individuals should consult with a healthcare professional before using ashwagandha supplements. It's important to use ashwagandha under the guidance of a healthcare professional and to discontinue use if any adverse effects occur.

Astragalus:

Definition: Astragalus, scientifically known as Astragalus membranaceus, is a flowering plant native to China and Mongolia but also found in other parts of Asia. It has been used for centuries in traditional Chinese medicine for its potential health benefits, particularly for its immune-enhancing properties.

Ingredients: Astragalus root contains various bioactive compounds, including polysaccharides, saponins (such as astragalosides), flavonoids, and amino acids. These compounds are believed to contribute to the herb's medicinal properties, including its potential as an adaptogen, immunomodulator, and anti-inflammatory agent.

How to Prepare: Astragalus is typically consumed as a powdered root, herbal tea, tincture, or in supplement form (such as capsules or tablets). To make tea, dried astragalus root slices are simmered in water for several minutes before being strained and consumed.

Dosage: The appropriate dosage of astragalus can vary depending on factors such as age, health status, and the specific preparation being used. It's important to follow the recommended dosage on the product label or consult with a qualified herbalist or healthcare professional for personalized guidance.

How to Use: Astragalus powder, tea, tincture, or supplements are typically taken orally. It's often consumed to support immune function, promote vitality, and enhance overall well-being.

Side Effects: Astragalus is generally considered safe for most people when used in moderate amounts. However, some individuals may experience mild side effects such as gastrointestinal upset or allergic reactions. It may also interact with certain medications or have adverse effects in individuals with certain health conditions, such as autoimmune diseases or diabetes. Pregnant or breastfeeding individuals should consult with a healthcare professional before using astragalus supplements. It's important to use astragalus under the guidance of a healthcare professional and to discontinue use if any adverse effects occur.

Black Cohosh:

Definition: Black cohosh, scientifically known as Actaea racemosa (formerly Cimicifuga racemosa), is a perennial herb native to North America. It has a long history of use in traditional Native American medicine and later in folk medicine for its potential health benefits, particularly for women's health.

Ingredients: Black cohosh root contains various bioactive compounds, including triterpene glycosides (such as actein and cimicifugoside), phenolic acids, and flavonoids. These compounds are believed to contribute to the herb's medicinal properties, including its potential as a hormone-balancing agent and its ability to relieve menopausal symptoms.

How to Prepare: Black cohosh is typically consumed as a powdered root, herbal tea, tincture, or in supplement form (such as capsules or tablets). To make tea, dried black cohosh root is steeped in hot water for several minutes before being strained and consumed.

Dosage: The appropriate dosage of black cohosh can vary depending on factors such as age, health status, and the specific preparation being used. It's important to follow the recommended dosage on the product label or consult with a qualified herbalist or healthcare professional for personalized guidance.

How to Use: Black cohosh powder, tea, tincture, or supplements are typically taken orally. It's often used by women to support hormonal balance, relieve menopausal symptoms such as hot flashes and night sweats, and promote overall well-being.

Side Effects: Black cohosh is generally considered safe for most people when used in moderate amounts. However, some individuals may experience mild side effects such as gastrointestinal upset or allergic reactions. It may also interact with certain medications or have adverse effects in individuals with certain health conditions, such as liver disease or hormone-sensitive conditions. Pregnant or breastfeeding individuals should consult with a healthcare professional before using black cohosh supplements. It's important to use black cohosh under the guidance of a healthcare professional and to discontinue use if any adverse effects occur.

Hydrangea:

Definition: Hydrangea, scientifically known as Hydrangea arborescens, is a flowering shrub native to North America. It has been used traditionally in herbal medicine for its potential diuretic and anti-inflammatory properties.

Ingredients: Hydrangea contains several bioactive compounds, including saponins, flavonoids, and glycosides. These compounds are believed to contribute to the herb's medicinal properties, including its potential as a diuretic, kidney tonic, and anti-inflammatory agent.

How to Prepare: Hydrangea root is typically prepared and consumed as an herbal tea or tincture. To make tea, dried hydrangea root is steeped in hot water for several minutes before being strained and consumed. Tinctures are prepared by steeping the root in alcohol or vinegar to extract its active compounds.

Dosage: The appropriate dosage of hydrangea can vary depending on factors such as age, health status, and the specific preparation being used. It's important to follow the recommended dosage on the product label or consult with a qualified herbalist or healthcare professional for personalized guidance.

How to Use: Hydrangea tea or tincture is typically taken orally. It's important to use hydrangea products as directed and to discontinue use if any adverse effects occur.

Side Effects: Hydrangea is generally considered safe for most people when used in moderate amounts. However, some individuals may experience digestive upset or allergic reactions. It may also interact with certain medications or have adverse effects in individuals with certain health conditions. It's important to use hydrangea under the guidance of a healthcare professional and to discontinue use if any adverse effects occur.

Irish Moss:

Definition: Irish Moss, scientifically known as Chondrus crispus, is a species of red algae or seaweed native to the Atlantic coastlines of Europe and North America. It has been used for centuries in traditional Irish and Scottish cuisine, as well as in herbal medicine.

Ingredients: Irish Moss is rich in various nutrients, including iodine, sulfur compounds, vitamins (such as vitamin A, vitamin K, and vitamin B12), minerals (including calcium, magnesium, potassium, and sodium), and polysaccharides (such as carrageenan). These nutrients are believed to contribute to the herb's potential health benefits.

How to Prepare: Irish Moss is typically prepared by soaking it in water to rehydrate and soften it before use. It can be added to soups, stews, smoothies, desserts, and other dishes as a thickening agent or nutritional supplement.

Dosage: The appropriate dosage of Irish Moss can vary depending on factors such as age, health status, and the specific preparation being used. It's important to follow recipes or guidelines for culinary use and to consult with a healthcare professional for guidance on using Irish Moss as a dietary supplement.

How to Use: Irish Moss can be used in culinary applications to add thickness and nutritional value to dishes. It can also be consumed as a dietary supplement in the form of capsules, powders, or extracts.

Side Effects: Irish Moss is generally considered safe for most people when consumed in moderate amounts as part of a balanced diet. However, some individuals may be allergic to seaweed or carrageenan, a compound found in Irish Moss that is used as a food additive. It's important to discontinue use if any adverse effects occur and to consult with a healthcare professional if you have any concerns.

Irish Sea Moss:

Definition: Irish Sea Moss is a term often used interchangeably with Irish Moss, referring to the same species of red algae, Chondrus crispus. It's harvested from the rocky shores of the Atlantic coastlines of Europe and North America.

Ingredients: Irish Sea Moss shares the same nutritional profile as Irish Moss, containing iodine, vitamins, minerals, and polysaccharides. It's valued for its potential health benefits, including supporting thyroid function, boosting immune health, and promoting digestion.

How to Prepare: Irish Sea Moss is prepared in the same way as Irish Moss, by soaking it in water to rehydrate and soften it before use. It can be used in culinary applications or consumed as a dietary supplement.

Dosage: The dosage of Irish Sea Moss depends on the form and intended use. As a dietary supplement, it's important to follow the recommended dosage on the product label or consult with a healthcare professional for personalized guidance.

How to Use: Irish Sea Moss can be used in various culinary applications, including soups, smoothies, desserts, and sauces. It can also be consumed as a dietary supplement in the form of capsules, powders, or extracts.

Side Effects: Similar to Irish Moss, Irish Sea Moss is generally considered safe for most people when consumed in moderate amounts. However, individuals with seaweed allergies or sensitivities to carrageenan should exercise caution. It's important to discontinue use if any adverse effects occur and to consult with a healthcare professional if you have any concerns.

Lymphalin:

Definition: Lymphalin is a herbal supplement formulated to support lymphatic system health. The lymphatic system plays a crucial role in immune function and waste removal in the body, and Lymphalin is designed to promote its proper function.

Ingredients: Lymphalin typically contains a blend of herbs and botanical extracts known for their traditional use in supporting lymphatic system health. Common ingredients may include cleavers, red clover, echinacea, burdock root, and calendula, among others.

How to Prepare: Lymphalin is usually available in capsule or liquid form. Capsules are taken orally with water, while liquid forms may be mixed with water or juice before consumption. It's important to follow the recommended dosage on the product label.

Dosage: The appropriate dosage of Lymphalin can vary depending on the specific product and individual needs. It's important to follow the recommended dosage on the product label or consult with a healthcare professional for personalized guidance.

How to Use: Lymphalin capsules are typically taken orally with water, while liquid forms may be mixed with water or juice before consumption. It's often recommended to take Lymphalin on an empty stomach for optimal absorption.

Side Effects: Lymphalin is generally considered safe for most people when used as directed. However, some individuals may experience mild side effects such as gastrointestinal discomfort or allergic reactions to certain ingredients. It's important to consult with a healthcare provider before starting any new supplement regimen, especially if you have underlying health conditions or are taking medications.

THE END